C000138051

Vibrators

100 of the best vibrators in the world

HarperCollins*Publishers*

HarperCollins*Publishers*
77–85 Fulham Palace Road,
Hammersmith, London W6 8JB
www.harpercollins.co.uk

First published by HarperCollins 2007

Copyright © Gavin Griffiths 2007
Photography by Paul Blundell
All images © Gavin Griffiths 2007

The Author asserts the moral right to
be identified as the author of this work

A catalogue record for this book
is available from the British Library

ISBN-13 978 0 00 726148 2
ISBN-10 0 00 726148 2

Design by Naomi Maister
Set in Helvetica

Printed and bound in Thailand by Imago

All rights reserved. No part of this publication may be
reproduced, stored in a retrieval system, or transmitted,
in any form or by any means, electronic, mechanical,
photocopying, recording or otherwise, without the prior
permission of the publishers.

Dedicated to Sarah, Naomi, Alyson, The Lauras G & D,
Mark, Andrea, Matthew, Simon, Jen, Clara, Hewitt & Dolly

Contents

Introduction

Many think that the vibrator is a new phenomenon, a symbol of the low moral mores of the sexed-up age in which we live. It's been reported that as many as 22% of adults in the developed world now own a vibrator. So where did this unbridled rampant pleasure-seeking suddenly come from? Has our decadent 'have it now' culture and half a century of female empowerment finally collided to create a world so dominated by the quest for sexual gratification that even our supermarkets are selling sex aids?

Historical evidence tells us that the only thing that has changed over the years is the media's coverage of the topic. It's clear that the origins of the vibrator are as ancient as mankind itself. Recently archaeologists unearthed a highly polished phallus in a cave in Germany dating back 28,000 years that they believe was used as a prehistoric dildo. How comforting to imagine our distant cave dwelling antecedents having a quiet night in with a bottle of Chablis and something special to spice up the old marital bed.

And we only have to fast forward twenty six millennia where we find Cleopatra who was said to have used a box of buzzing bees to pleasure herself on nights when Mark Anthony was away attempting to vanquish Persia. In our more recent history, 19th-century sexually frustrated women didn't have the benefit of a sex shop on every high street and instead were regularly diagnosed with 'hysteria', the cure for which was a visit to the doctor where manual relief was administered for a lucrative fee. Ever pragmatic and with an eye for business, the Victorian medical profession soon discovered that women could be more easily cured if a mechanical device was used to do the job and this was the inspiration for the modern day vibrator.

Today there are thousands available. Some are visually stunning design classics that would make Philippe Starck jealous, while others adopt function over form and would probably make Starck slightly embarrassed. There are those handcrafted from solid gold, and some that fix onto the end of an electric toothbrush.

This book is a collection of our 100 favourites on the market today – beautiful and shocking by turn, revolutionary to female pleasure and compelling to observe – they come in all manner of shape, size and functionality from the popular Thruster (page 125) and the comic Duckie (page 23) to the bizarre Cone (page 15). Each one has been rigorously tested by a highly discerning panel of judges from the *Scarlet* team. What's your favourite? Take your pick, and remember there's no shame – we've been playing with sex toys for 28,000 years!

G Griffiths
Publisher and founder of *Scarlet* magazine

Octopus Massager

Appearance	●●●●○
Originality	●●●●●
Subtlety	●●●●○
Portability	●●●●○
Orgasmability	●●○○○

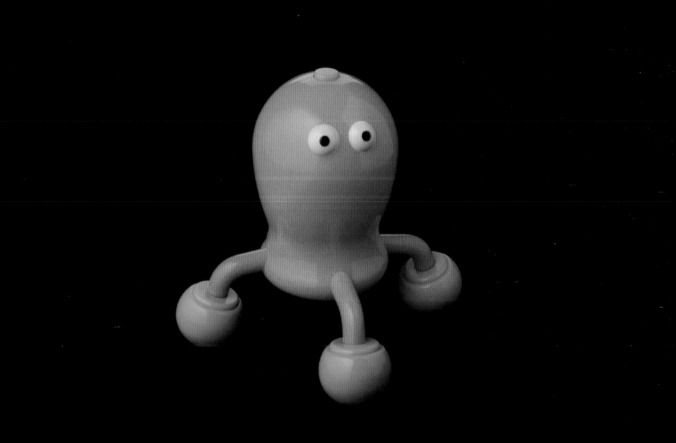

Sea Foam

Appearance	●●●●○
Originality	●●●●●
Subtlety	●●●●○
Portability	●●●●○
Orgasmability	●●●○○

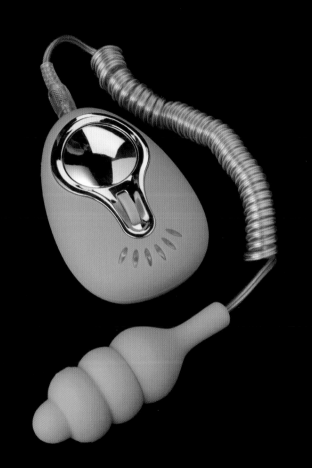

Iris

Appearance	●●●●●
Originality	●●●○○
Subtlety	●●●○○
Portability	●●○○○
Orgasmability	●●●●●

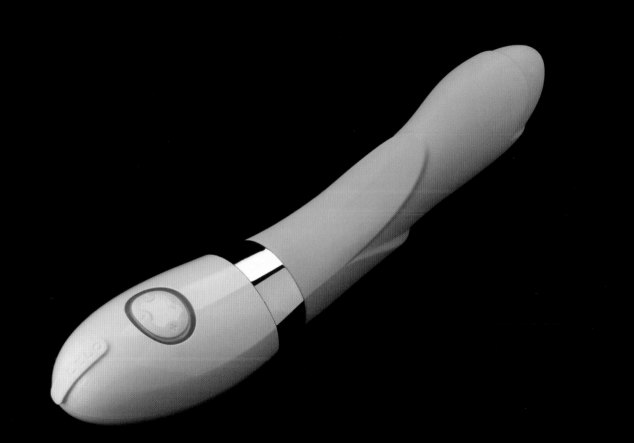

I-gasm

Appearance	●●●○○
Originality	●●●●●
Subtlety	●●●●○
Portability	●●●●○
Orgasmability	●●○○○

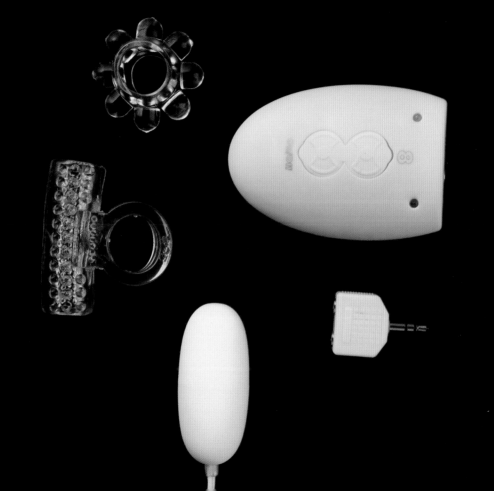

Smartvibe GII

Appearance	●●●○○
Originality	●●●●○
Subtlety	●○○○○
Portability	●●○○○
Orgasmability	●●●●●

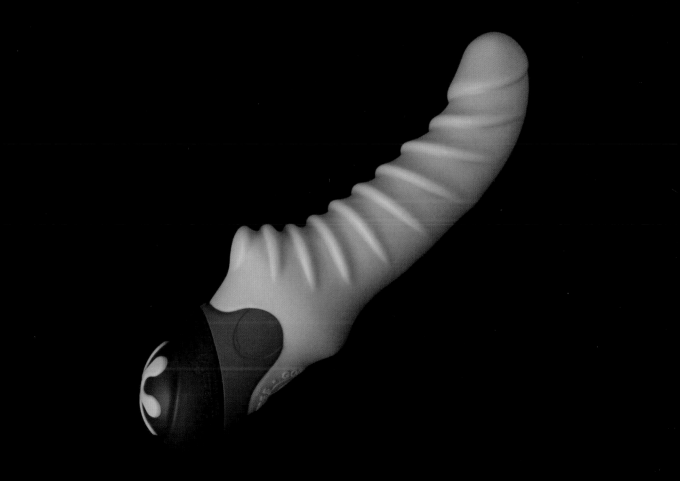

Promise

Appearance	●●○○○
Originality	●●○○○
Subtlety	●●●●○
Portability	●●●○○
Orgasmability	●●○○○

Copper Tantus

Appearance	●●●○○
Originality	●●○○○
Subtlety	●●●○○
Portability	●●●●○
Orgasmability	●●○○○

Stubby

Appearance	●●●●○
Originality	●●●●○
Subtlety	●●○○○
Portability	●●●○○
Orgasmability	●●●●○

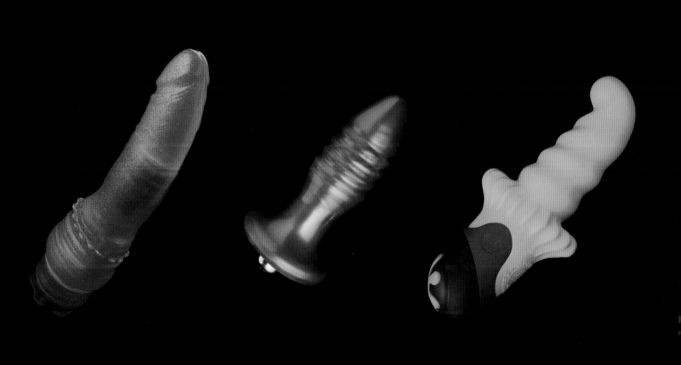

The Cone

Appearance	●●●●●
Originality	●●●●●
Subtlety	●○○○○
Portability	○○○○○
Orgasmability	●●●●○

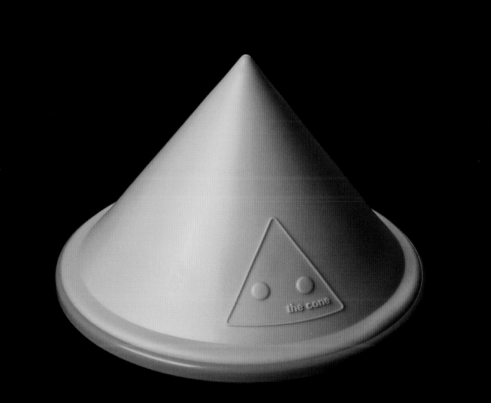

the cone

Lily

Appearance	●●●●○
Originality	●●●●●
Subtlety	●●●●●
Portability	●●●●●
Orgasmability	●●●●●

Yva

Appearance	●●●●●
Originality	●●●●●
Subtlety	●●●●●
Portability	●●●●●
Orgasmability	●●●●●

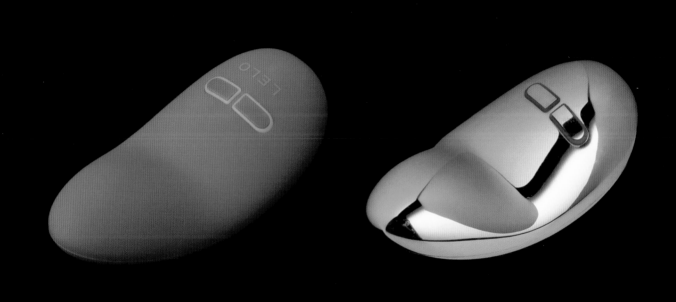

Miyakodori

Appearance	●●○○○
Originality	●●●●○
Subtlety	●●●●○
Portability	●●●●○
Orgasmability	●○○○○

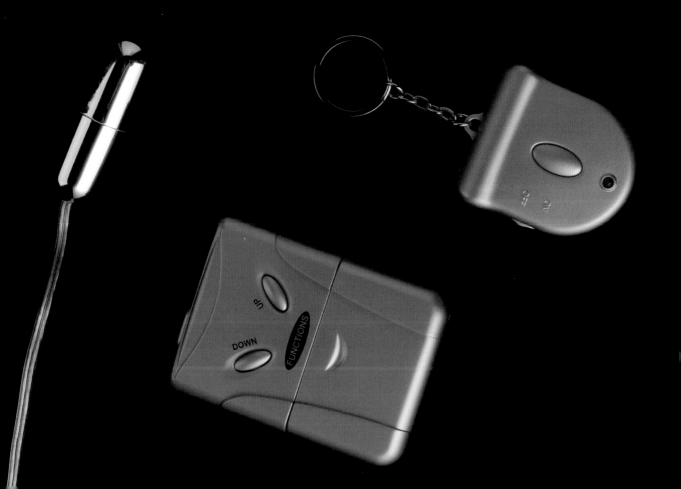

Ideal

Appearance	●●●●○
Originality	●●●●●
Subtlety	●●●○○
Portability	●●○○○
Orgasmability	●●●●○

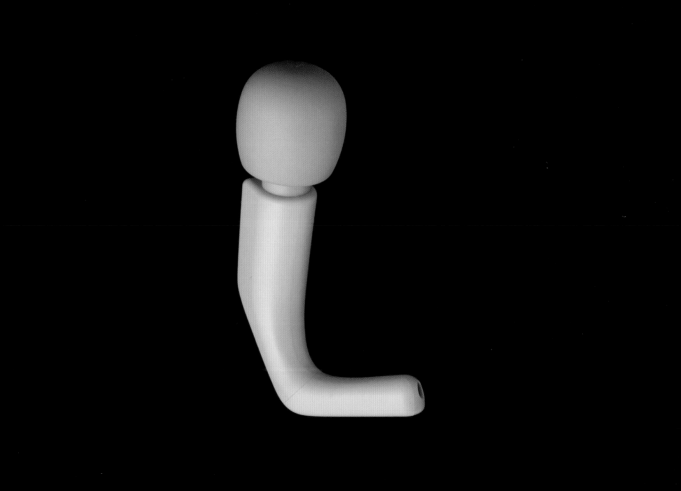

I Rub My Duckie

Appearance	●●●○○
Originality	●●●●●
Subtlety	●●●●○
Portability	●●●○○
Orgasmability	●●●○○

Duckie, Paris Edition

Appearance	●●●●○
Originality	●●●●●
Subtlety	●●●○○
Portability	●●●○○
Orgasmability	●●●○○

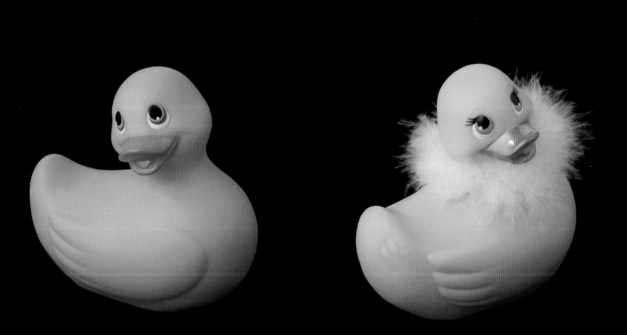

Duchess

Appearance	●●●●○
Originality	●●○○○
Subtlety	●●○○○
Portability	●●○○○
Orgasmability	●●●●○

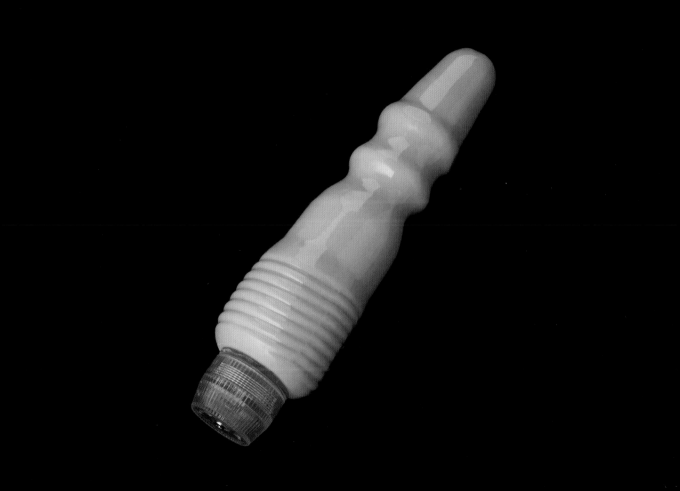

Mellow Yellow

Appearance	●●○○○
Originality	●●●●●
Subtlety	●●○○○
Portability	●○○○○
Orgasmability	●●●○○

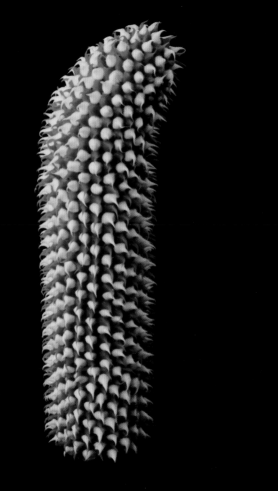

Liberte

Appearance	●●●●○
Originality	●●●●○
Subtlety	●●●○○
Portability	●●○○○
Orgasmability	●●●●○

Twist 'n' Shake

Appearance	●●●○○
Originality	●●○○○
Subtlety	●○○○○
Portability	●●○○○
Orgasmability	●●●●○

Royal Sceptre

Appearance	●●○○○
Originality	●●○○○
Subtlety	●●●○○
Portability	●●●○○
Orgasmability	●●●○○

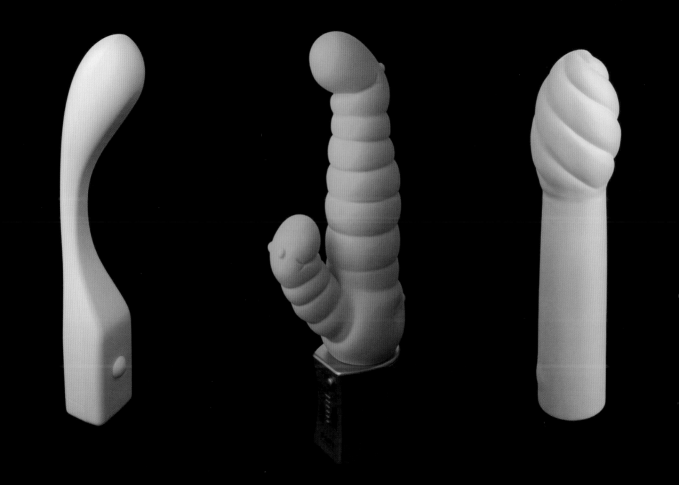

Adonis

Appearance	●●○○○
Originality	●●●●○
Subtlety	●●○○○
Portability	●●○○○
Orgasmability	●●●○○

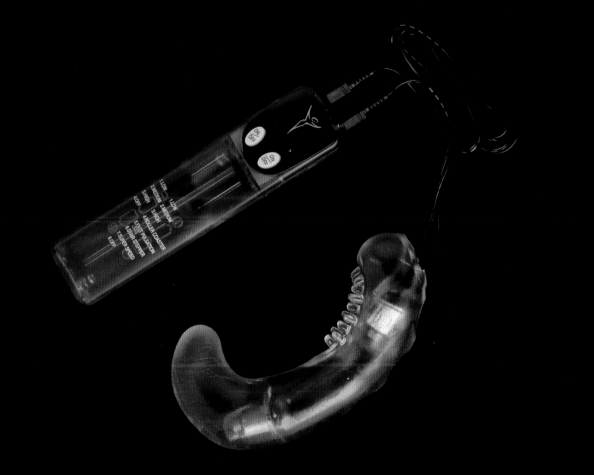

Mini Flexo Pleaser

Appearance	●●●●○
Originality	●●●●●
Subtlety	●●●○○
Portability	●●●○○
Orgasmability	●●●○○

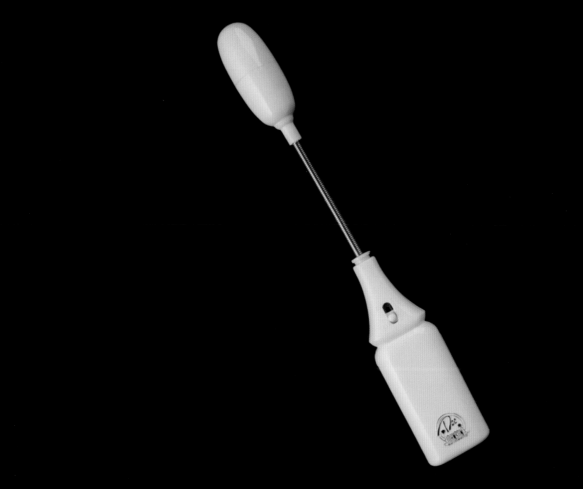

Sinnflut

Appearance	●●●●○
Originality	●●●●○
Subtlety	●○○○○
Portability	●○○○○
Orgasmability	●●●●●

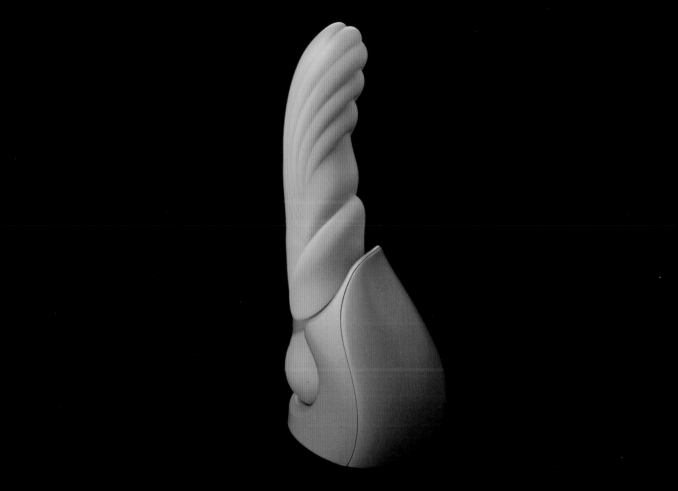

Omibod

Appearance	●●○○○
Originality	●●○○○
Subtlety	●●●○○
Portability	●●○○○
Orgasmability	●●●●○

Mary Mermaid

Appearance	●●●○○
Originality	●●●○○
Subtlety	●●○○○
Portability	●●○○○
Orgasmability	●●●●○

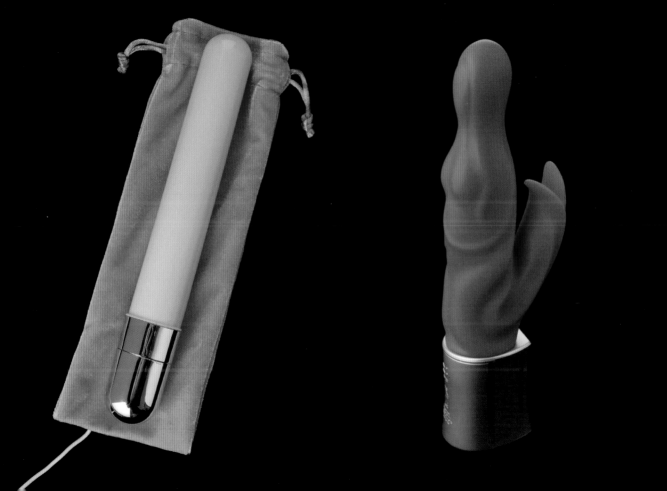

Pleasure Bullet

Appearance	●○○○○
Originality	●●●●○
Subtlety	●●●○○
Portability	●●●●○
Orgasmability	●●●○○

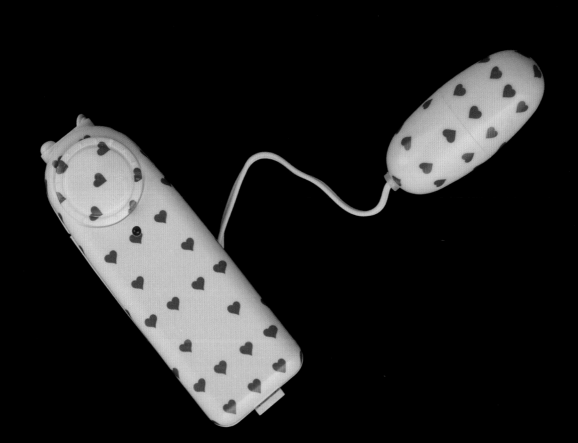

The Charm

Appearance	●●●●○
Originality	●●●●○
Sublety	●●●○○
Portability	●●○○○
Orgasmability	●●●●○

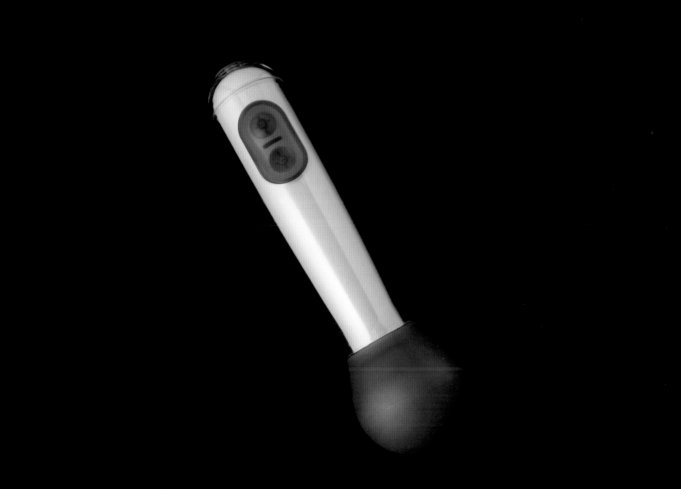

Vibrating Clit Massager

Appearance	●○○○○
Originality	●●●●○
Subtlety	●●○○○
Portability	●●○○○
Orgasmability	●●●●○

Erotic Butterfly

Appearance	●●○○○
Originality	●●●●○
Subtlety	●●○○○
Portability	●●●○○
Orgasmability	●●●○○

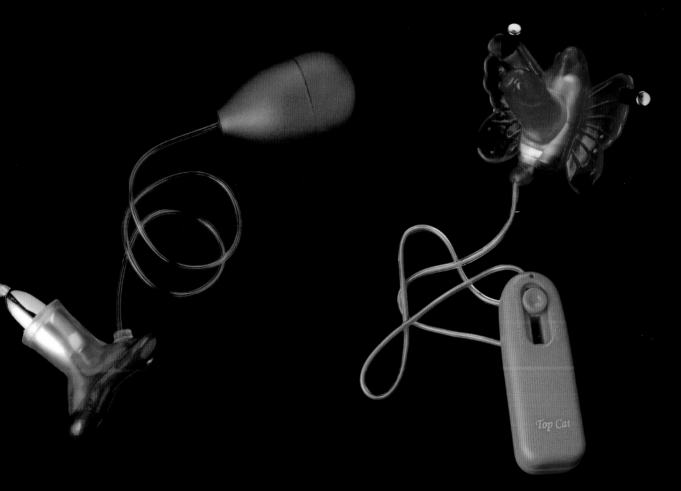

Mr Big

Appearance	●●●○○
Originality	●○○○○
Subtlety	●○○○○
Portability	●●○○○
Orgasmability	●●●●●

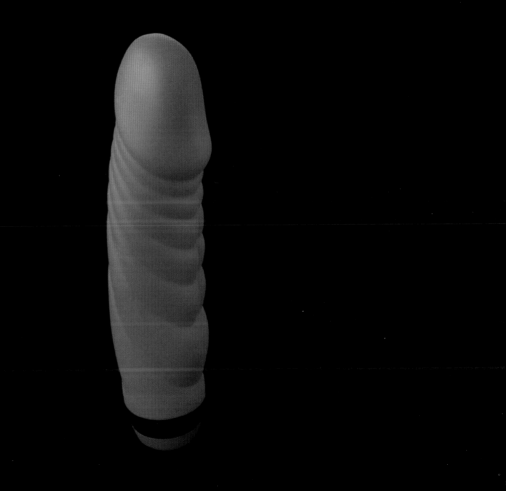

Devil's Tongue

Appearance	●●○○○
Originality	●●●●○
Subtlety	●●○○○
Portability	●●●○○
Orgasmability	●●○○○

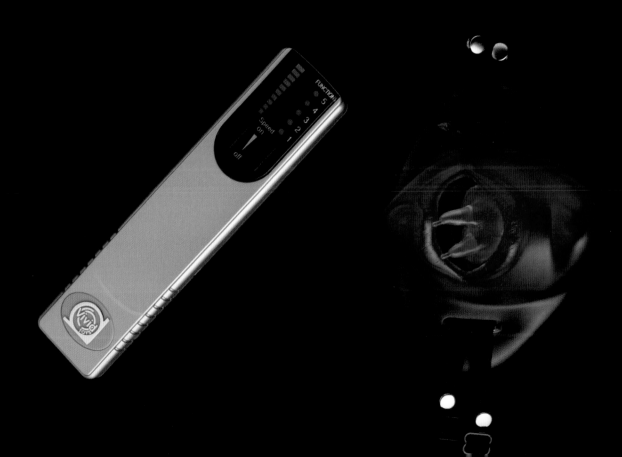

Flower Power

Appearance	●●●●○
Originality	●●●●●
Subtlety	●●●●●
Portability	●●●○○
Orgasmability	●●●○○

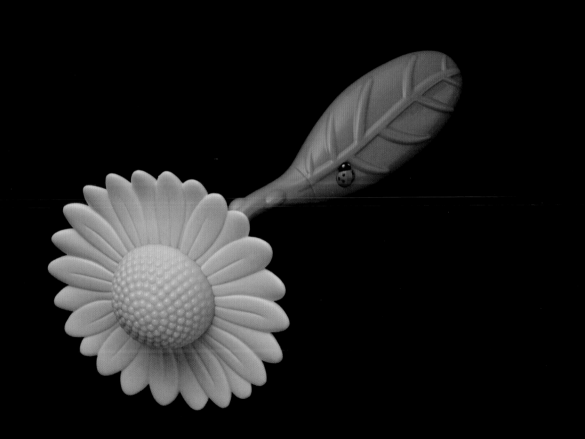

Monroe's Lips

Appearance	○○○○○
Originality	●●●○○
Subtlety	●●○○○
Portability	●●○○○
Orgasmability	●●●●○

Lucid Dreams, No. 14

Appearance	●●●●○
Originality	●●●○○
Sublety	●●○○○
Portability	●●○○○
Orgasmability	●●●●○

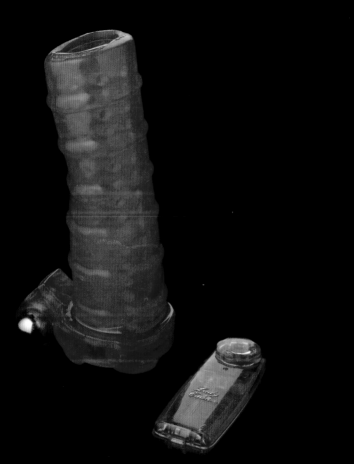
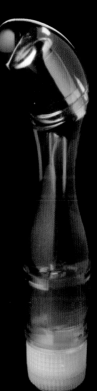

Laya Spot

Appearance	●●●●●
Originality	●●●●○
Subtlety	●●●●○
Portability	●●●●○
Orgasmability	●●●●●

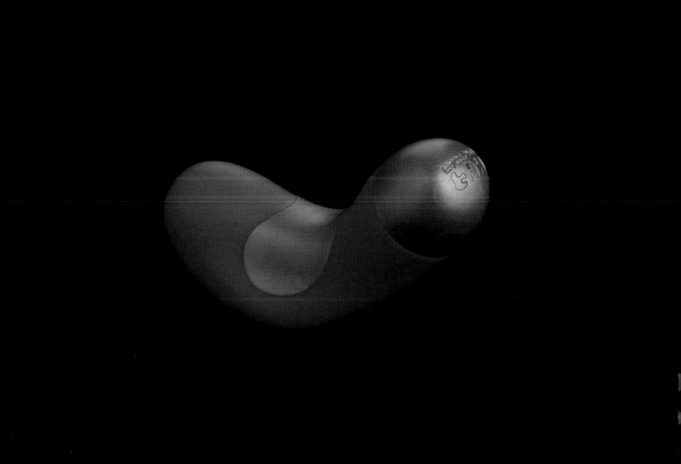

Japanese Extreme

Appearance	●○○○○
Originality	●●●●○
Subtlety	○○○○○
Portability	●○○○○
Orgasmability	●●●●○

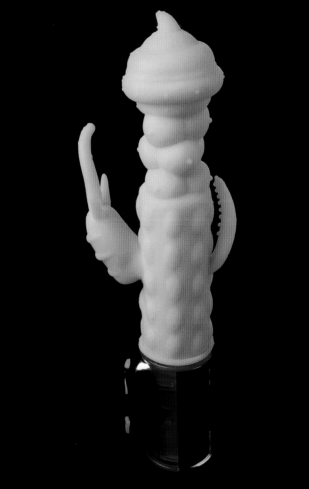

Long Neck Tortoise

Appearance	●●○○○
Originality	●●●●○
Subtlety	●●○○○
Portability	●●●○○
Orgasmability	●●●○○

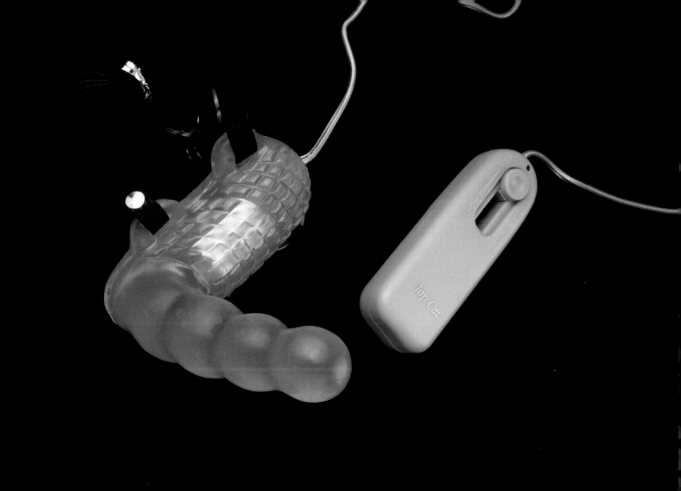

Jungle G Tiger

Appearance	●●●●○
Originality	●●●○○
Subtlety	●●○○○
Portability	●●●○○
Orgasmability	●●●●○

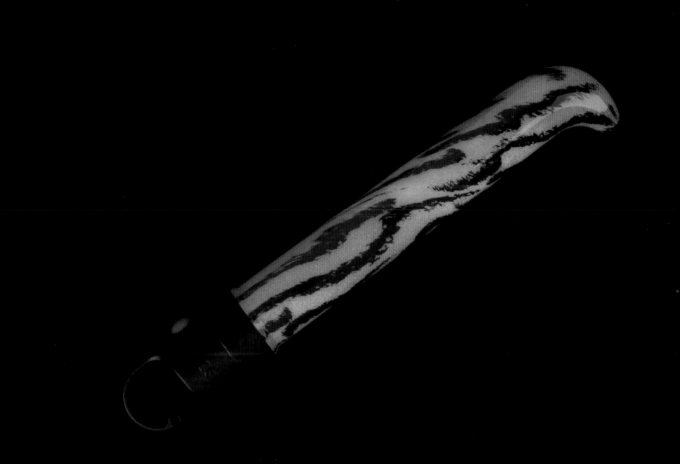

Mates Condom Ring

Appearance	●○○○○
Originality	●●●●○
Subtlety	●●○○○
Portability	●●●●○
Orgasmability	●●●●○

Maia

Appearance	●●●●○
Originality	●●●○○
Subtlety	●●●●●
Portability	●●●●●
Orgasmability	●●○○○

Thorn Bird

Appearance	●●○○○
Originality	●●○○○
Subtlety	●●○○○
Portability	●●●○○
Orgasmability	●●○○○

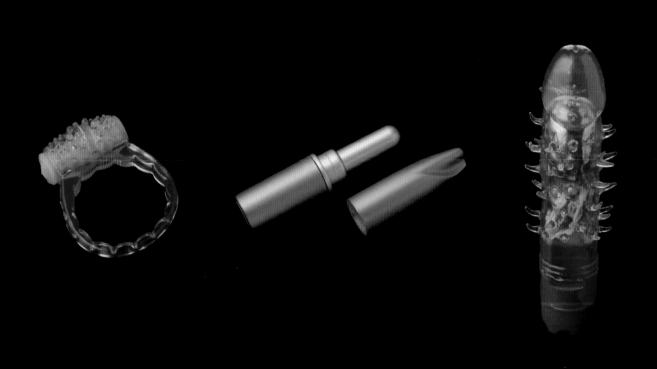

Pure Vibes

Appearance	●●●●○
Originality	●●○○○
Subtlety	●●○○○
Portability	●●○○○
Orgasmability	●●●●○

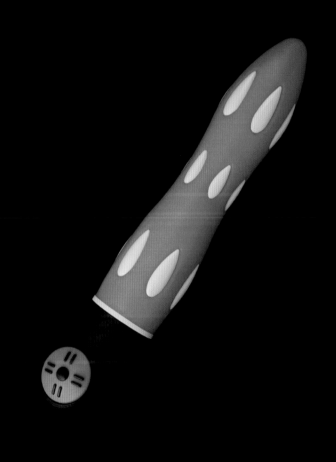

Retractable Heart

Appearance	●●●○○
Originality	●●●●○
Subtlety	●●●●○
Portability	●●●●○
Orgasmability	●●○○○

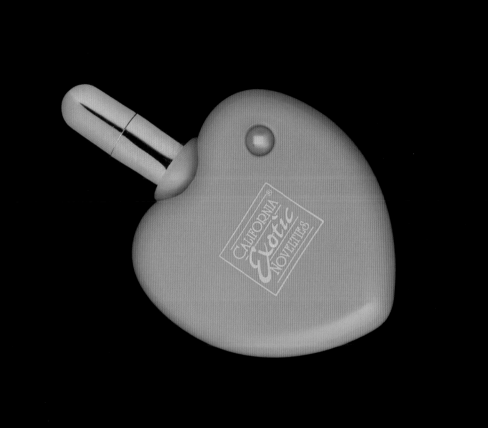

Vibral Whip

Appearance	●●●○○
Originality	●●●●●
Subtlety	●○○○○
Portability	●○○○○
Orgasmability	●○○○○

Elysia

Appearance	●●●●○
Originality	●●●○○
Subtlety	●●○○○
Portability	●●●●●
Orgasmability	●●○○○

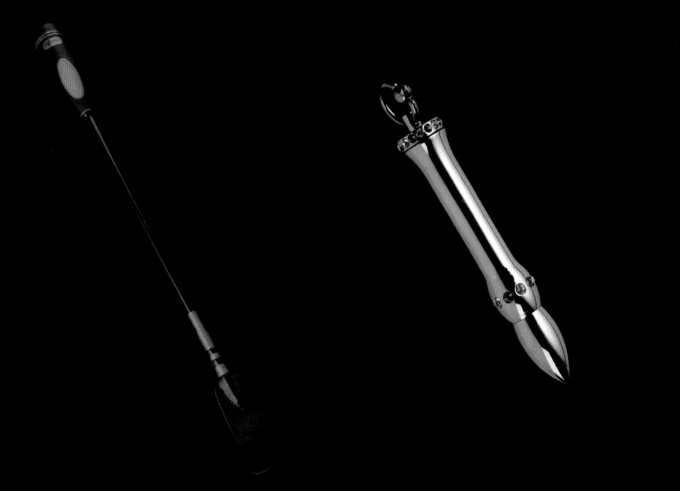

Red Tipped Crystal Ice Big Boss

Appearance	●●●●○
Originality	●●○○○
Subtlety	●○○○○
Portability	●●○○○
Orgasmability	●●●●●

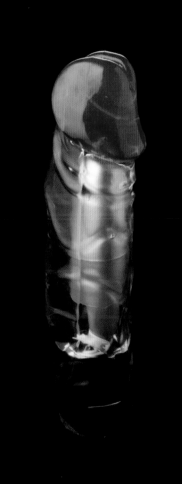

Royal Wizard

Appearance	●●●●○
Originality	●●●●○
Sublety	●●○○○
Portability	●●○○○
Orgasmability	●●●●○

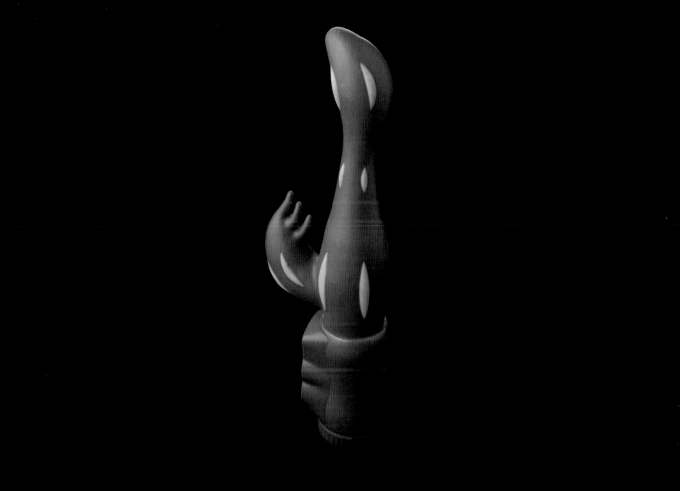

Madame Butterfly 2

Appearance	●○○○○
Originality	●●●●○
Subtlety	●○○○○
Portability	●○○○○
Orgasmability	●●●●○

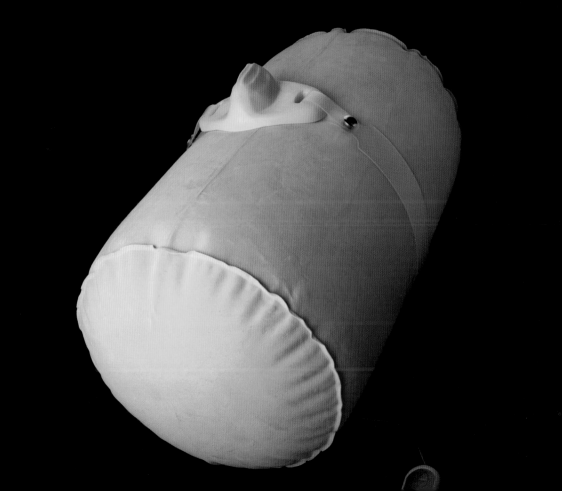

Mini Tongue

Appearance	●○○○○
Originality	●●●●●
Subtlety	●○○○○
Portability	●●●●○
Orgasmability	●●●○○

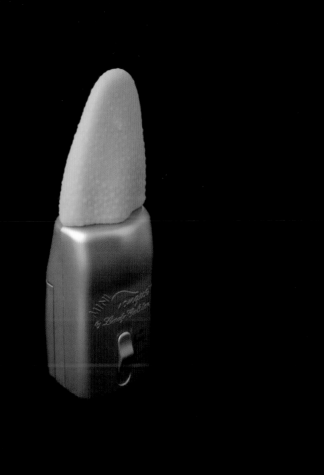

Flicker Mini

Appearance	●●○○○
Originality	●●○○○
Subtlety	●●○○○
Portability	●●●○○
Orgasmability	●●●○○

Tingle Tip

Appearance	●○○○○
Originality	●●●●○
Subtlety	●●●●●
Portability	●●●●●
Orgasmability	●●○○○

Smartvibe Watermelon

Appearance	●●●○○
Originality	●●●●○
Subtlety	●○○○○
Portability	●●○○○
Orgasmability	●●●●●

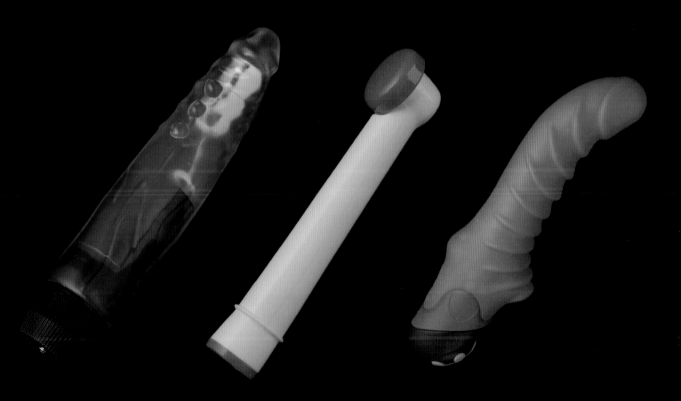

Rock Chick

Appearance	●●●○○
Originality	●●●●●
Subtlety	●●○○○
Portability	●●○○○
Orgasmability	●●●●○

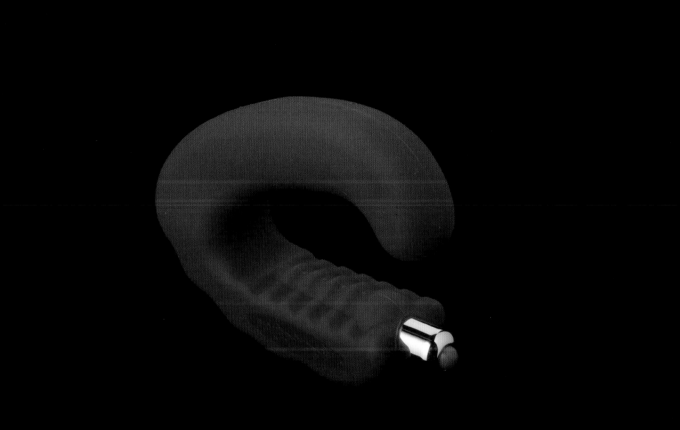

Magic Wand

Appearance	●●●●●
Originality	●●●●○
Subtlety	●●●●○
Portability	●●●○○
Orgasmability	●●●●○

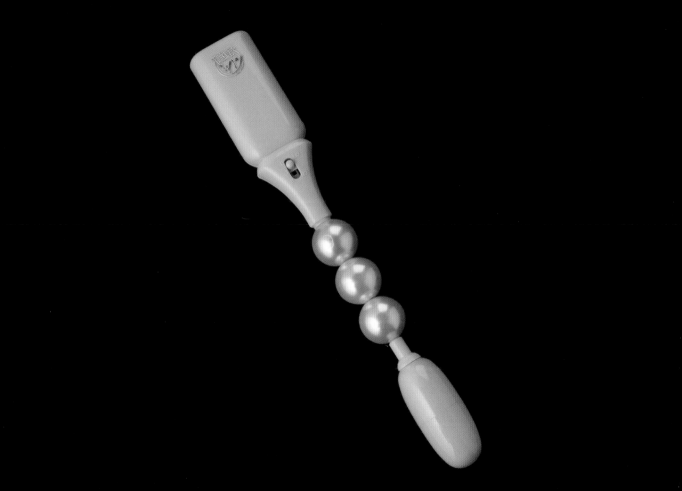

Let it Ride Dong

Appearance	●●●○○
Originality	●●●●○
Subtlety	●●●●○
Portability	●●○○○
Orgasmability	●●●●○

Waterplay

Appearance	●●○○○
Originality	●●○○○
Subtlety	●●●○○
Portability	●●●○○
Orgasmability	●●●●○

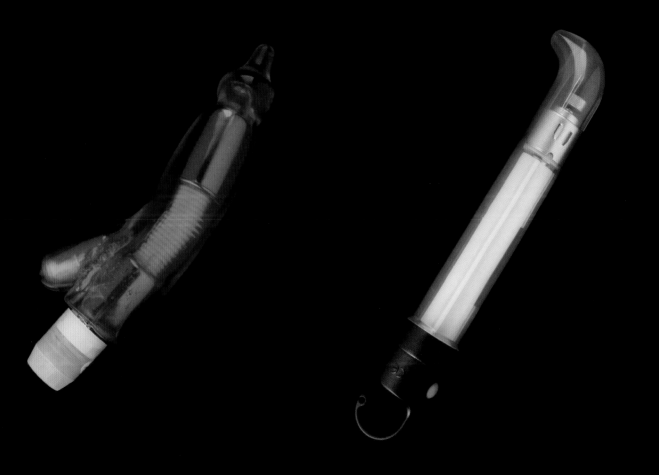

Portable Massager

Appearance	●●○○○
Originality	●○○○○
Subtlety	●●○○○
Portability	●●●○○
Orgasmability	●●●○○

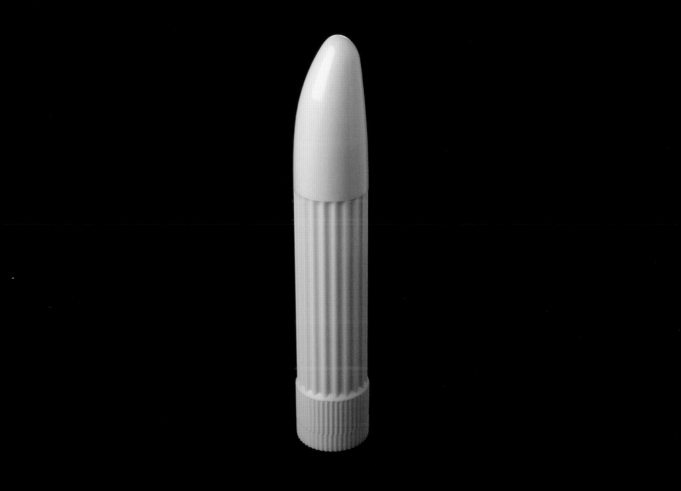

Rabbit Elite

Appearance	●●○○○
Originality	●●○○○
Subtlety	●○○○○
Portability	●●○○○
Orgasmability	●●●●●

Clone Boy*

Appearance	
Originality	
Subtlety	
Portability	
Orgasmability	

*all catagory scores will vary according to appearance and dimensions of original model

Incognito Mascara

Appearance	●●○○○
Originality	●●●●○
Subtlety	●●●●●
Portability	●●●●○
Orgasmability	●●○○○

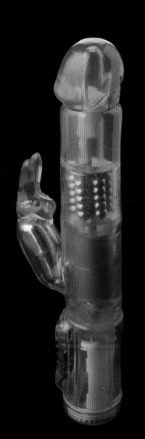
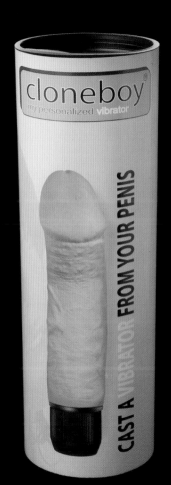
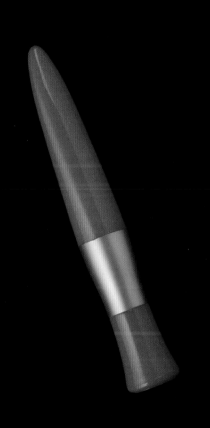

cloneboy
my personalized vibrator

CAST A VIBRATOR FROM YOUR PENIS

Little Gem

Appearance	●●●●●
Originality	●●●●●
Subtlety	●●●●●
Portability	●●○○○
Orgasmability	●●●●○

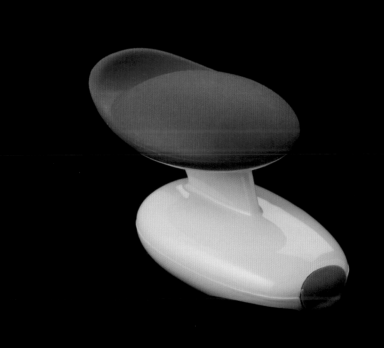

Wiggle Wand

Appearance	●●○○○
Originality	●●●●○
Subtlety	●●○○○
Portability	●●○○○
Orgasmability	●●●○○

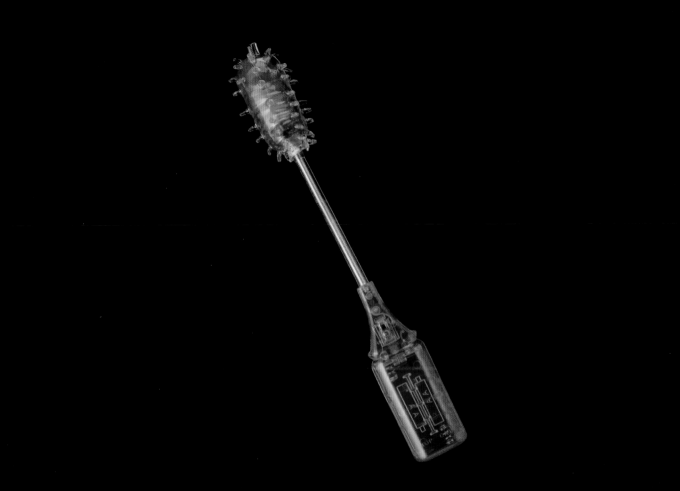

Ultime Personal Massager

Appearance	●●●●○
Originality	●●●●●
Subtlety	●●●●○
Portability	●●●○○
Orgasmability	●●●●○

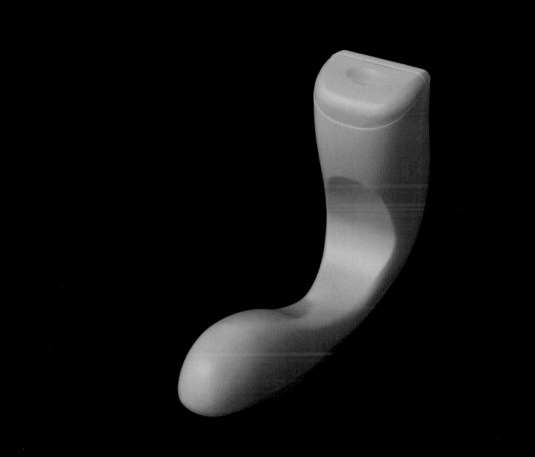

Bubblegum

Appearance	●●●○○
Originality	●●○○○
Subtlety	●○○○○
Portability	●●○○○
Orgasmability	●●●●○

Wireless Clit Climaxer

Appearance	●●○○○
Originality	●●●●○
Subtlety	●●○○○
Portability	●●●●○
Orgasmability	●●●●○

White Tantus

Appearance	●●●●○
Originality	●●○○○
Subtlety	●○○○○
Portability	●●○○○
Orgasmability	●●●○○

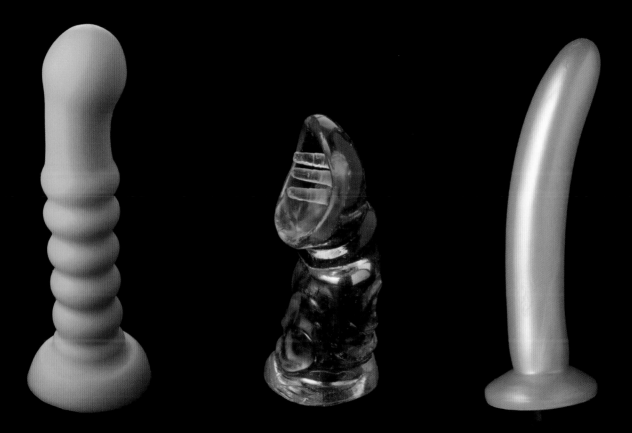

Luscious Lippy

Appearance	●●●○○
Originality	●●●●●
Subtlety	●●●●●
Portability	●●●●●
Orgasmability	●●○○○

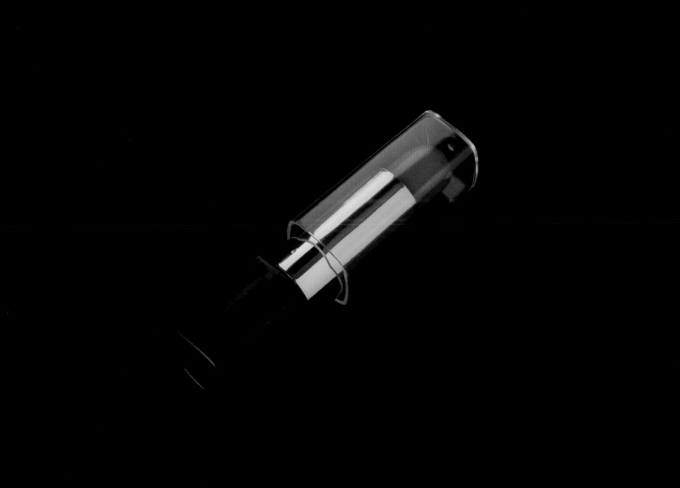

Lucid Dreams, No. 7

Appearance	●●●○○
Originality	●●●●○
Subtlety	●●●○○
Portability	●●●○○
Orgasmability	●●●○○

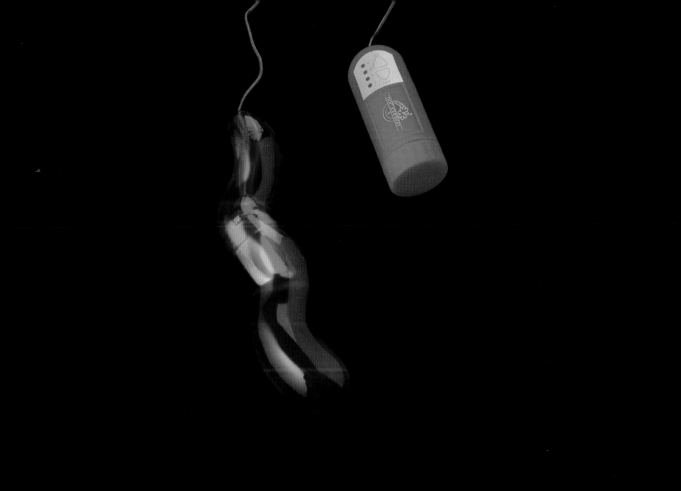

Go Go Stick

Appearance	●●●●●
Originality	●●●●○
Subtlety	●●●○○
Portability	●●○○○
Orgasmability	●●○○○

G-Spot Japex

Appearance	●○○○○
Originality	●●○○○
Subtlety	●○○○○
Portability	●●○○○
Orgasmability	●●●●○

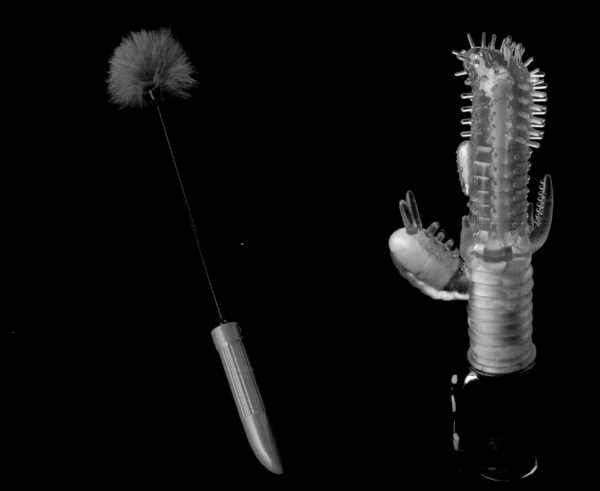

Dinky Ring

Appearance	●●●○○
Originality	●●●●○
Subtlety	●●●○○
Portability	●●●●●
Orgasmability	●●●●○

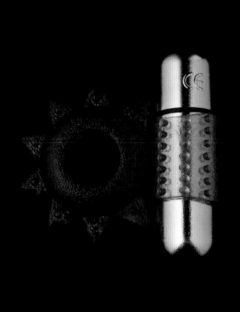

Gigolo

Appearance	●●●○○
Originality	●●○○○
Subtlety	●●○○○
Portability	●●○○○
Orgasmability	●●●●○

Glow-in-the-Dark Jelly Penis

Appearance	●●○○○
Originality	●●○○○
Subtlety	●○○○○
Portability	●●○○○
Orgasmability	●●●●○

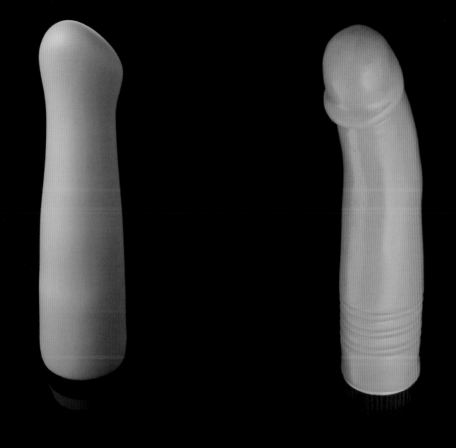

Wand

Appearance	●●●●○
Originality	●●●●●
Subtlety	●●●●○
Portability	●●●○○
Orgasmability	●●●●○

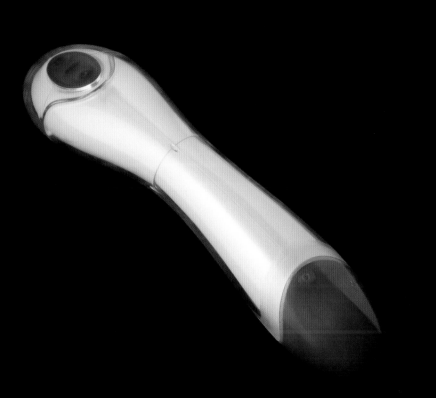

Knicker Critter

Appearance	●○○○○
Originality	●●●●●
Subtlety	●●●○○
Portability	●●●○○
Orgasmability	●●●●○

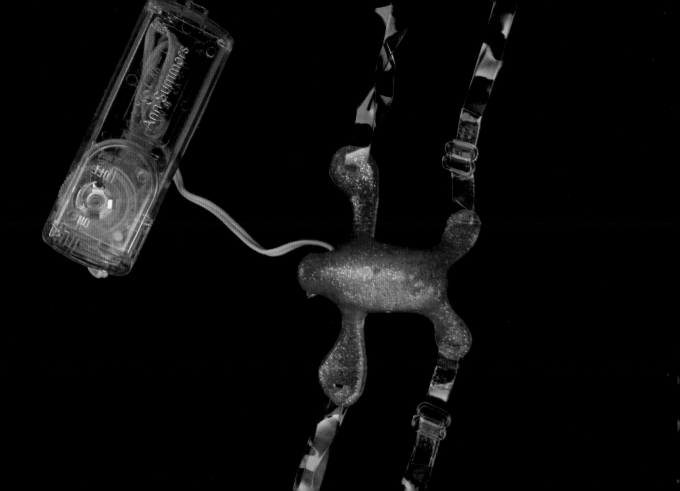

Freshvibes Mini

Appearance	●●●○○
Originality	●●○○○
Subtlety	●●○○○
Portability	●●●○○
Orgasmability	●●●○○

Goddess

Appearance	●●○○○
Originality	●○○○○
Subtlety	●●○○○
Portability	●●●○○
Orgasmability	●●●○○

Jenna's Curves

Appearance	●●●●○
Originality	●●●○○
Subtlety	●●●●○
Portability	●●●○○
Orgasmability	●●○○○

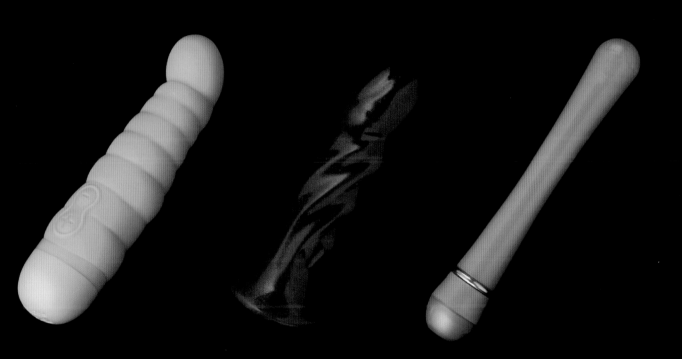

Little Chroma

Appearance	●●●●○
Originality	●●●○○
Subtlety	●●●●○
Portability	●●○○○
Orgasmability	●●●○○

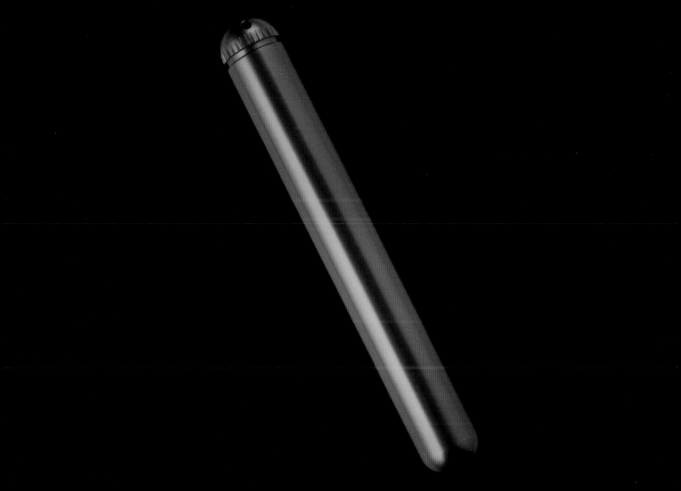

Tongue Joy

Appearance	●●●●○
Originality	●●●●●
Subtlety	●●●●●
Portability	●●●●●
Orgasmability	●●●●●

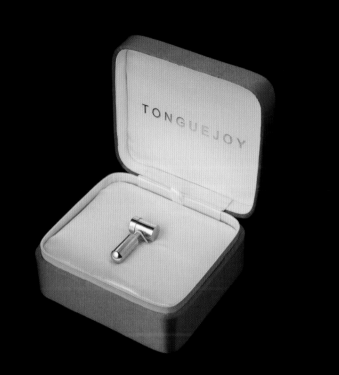

The Joy Stick

Appearance	●●●○○
Originality	●●●●○
Subtlety	●●○○○
Portability	●●○○○
Orgasmability	●●●○○

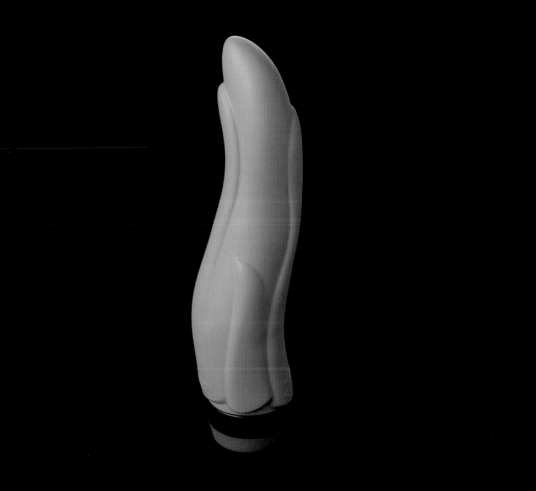

Cleopatra

Appearance	●●●○○
Originality	●●●●○
Subtlety	●●●●●
Portability	●●●●○
Orgasmability	●●●○○

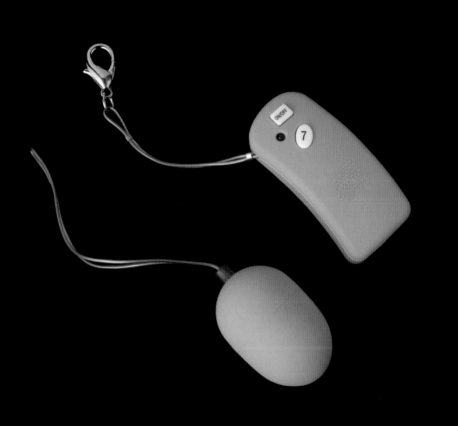

7" Smoothie

Appearance	●●○○○
Originality	●○○○○
Subtlety	●●○○○
Portability	●●●○○
Orgasmability	●●●○○

Royal Teaser

Appearance	●●●●○
Originality	●●●○○
Subtlety	●●●●○
Portability	●●●○○
Orgasmability	●●●○○

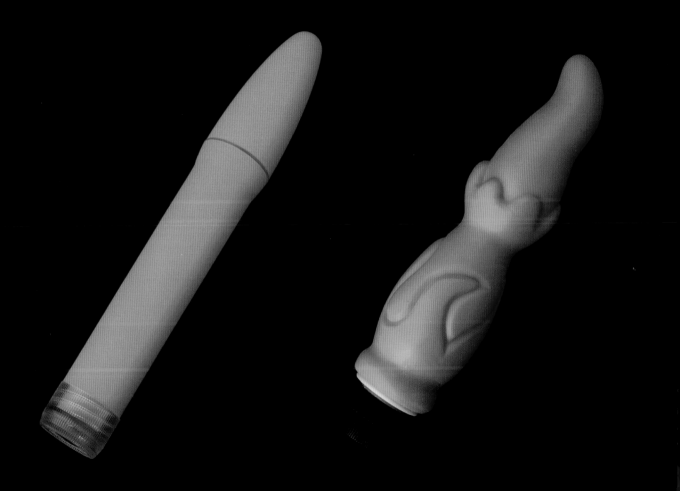

Ammunition for Love

Appearance	●●●●○
Originality	●●●○○
Subtlety	●●●●○
Portability	●●●●●
Orgasmability	●●●○○

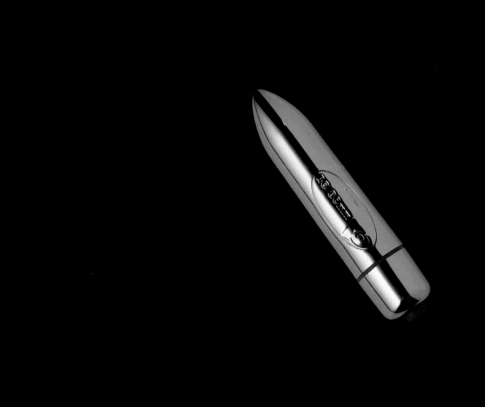

Gemini

Appearance	●●○○○
Originality	●●●●○
Subtlety	○○○○○
Portability	●○○○○
Orgasmability	●●●●○

The Thruster

Appearance	●●●○○
Originality	●●○○○
Subtlety	●○○○○
Portability	●●○○○
Orgasmability	●●●●●

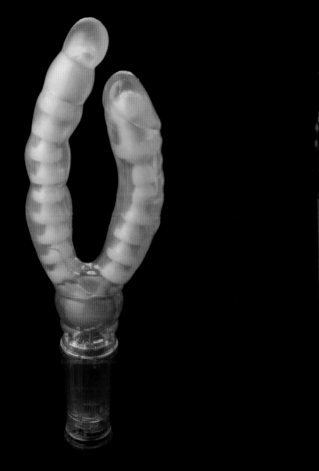
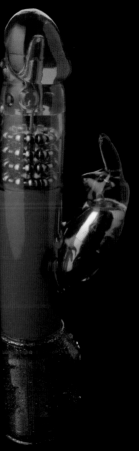

Double Play

Appearance	●●●○○
Originality	●●●○○
Subtlety	●●●●○
Portability	●●●●○
Orgasmability	●●●○○

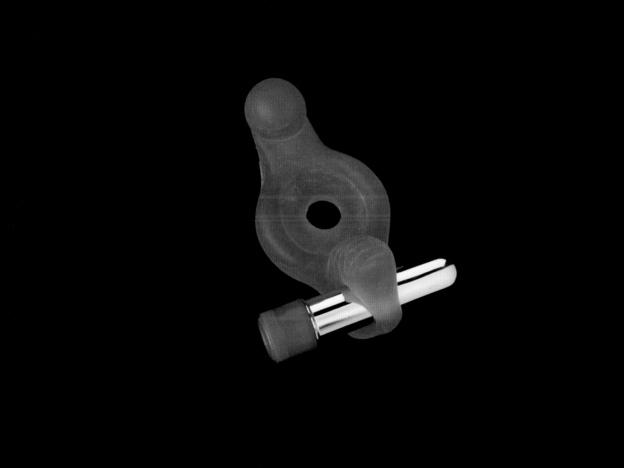

Ultra Seven

Appearance	●●●○○
Originality	●●●○○
Subtlety	●○○○○
Portability	●●○○○
Orgasmability	●●●●○

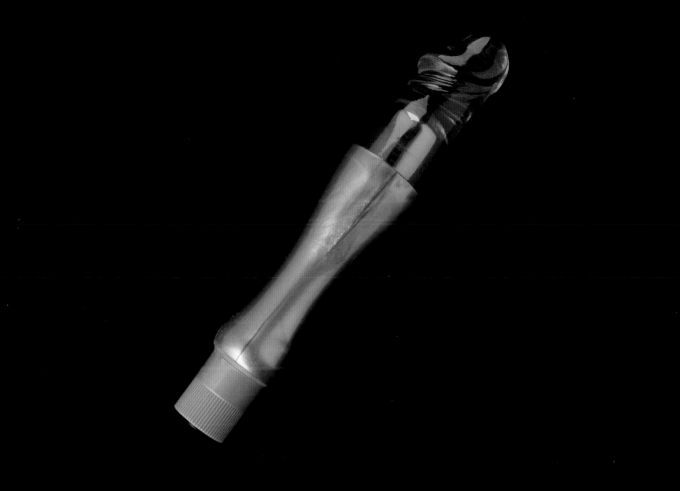

Dinky Rabbit

Appearance	●●●○○
Originality	●●●●●
Subtlety	●●●●○
Portability	●●●●●
Orgasmability	●●○○○

Dinky Mushroom

Appearance	●○○○○
Originality	●●●●○
Subtlety	●●●●○
Portability	●●●●●
Orgasmability	●●●○○

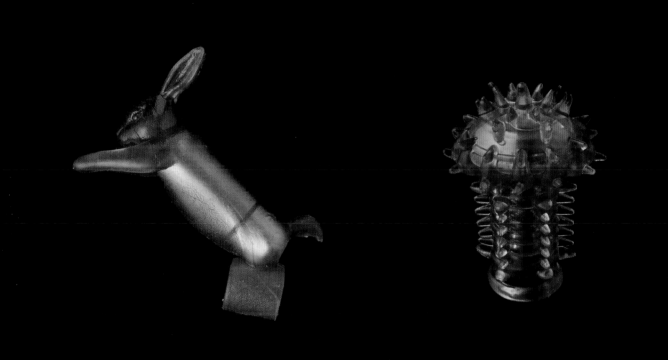

Pulsatron II

Appearance	●●●●○
Originality	●●●●○
Subtlety	●●●●○
Portability	●●●○○
Orgasmability	●●○○○

Sensual Curves

Appearance	●●○○○
Originality	●●●○○
Subtlety	●●○○○
Portability	●●●○○
Orgasmability	●●●○○

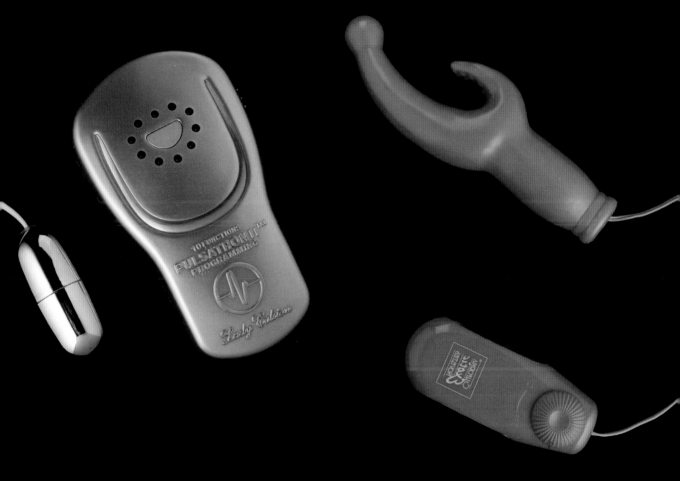

Silicone Vibro Ring

Appearance	●●○○○
Originality	●●●○○
Subtlety	●●○○○
Portability	●●●○○
Orgasmability	●●●●○

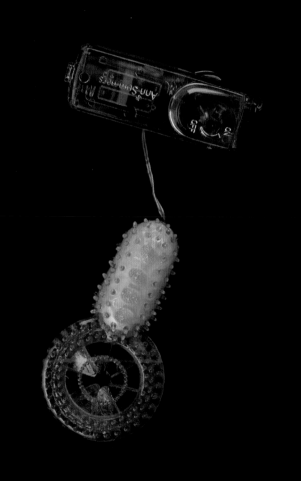

Zing Finger

Appearance	●●○○○
Originality	●●●●●
Subtlety	●●●○○
Portability	●●●○○
Orgasmability	●●●●●

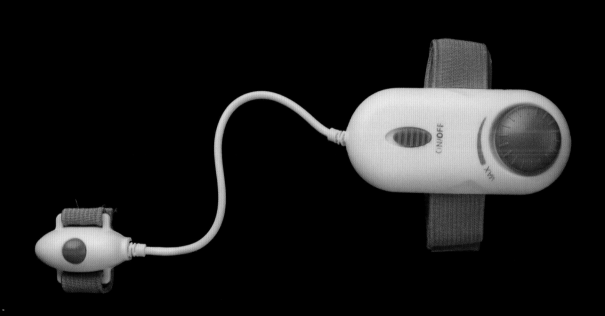

Pleasure Probe

Appearance	●●●○○
Originality	●●●●○
Subtlety	●●●○○
Portability	●●○○○
Orgasmability	●●●●○

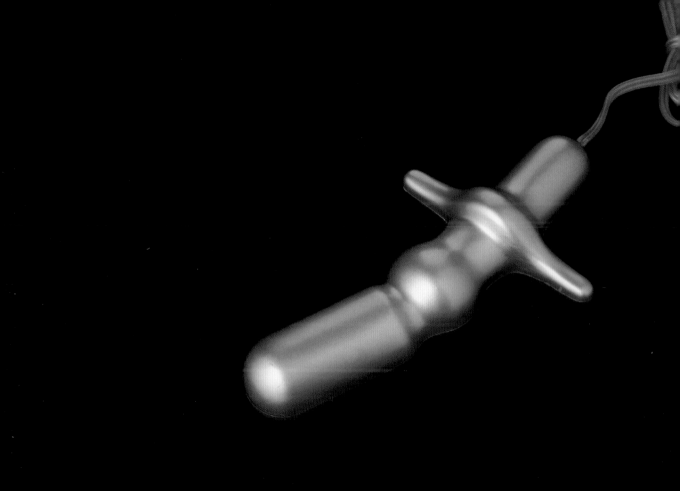

The Gipsy II

Appearance	●●○○○
Originality	●●●●○
Subtlety	●○○○○
Portability	●●○○○
Orgasmability	●●●○○

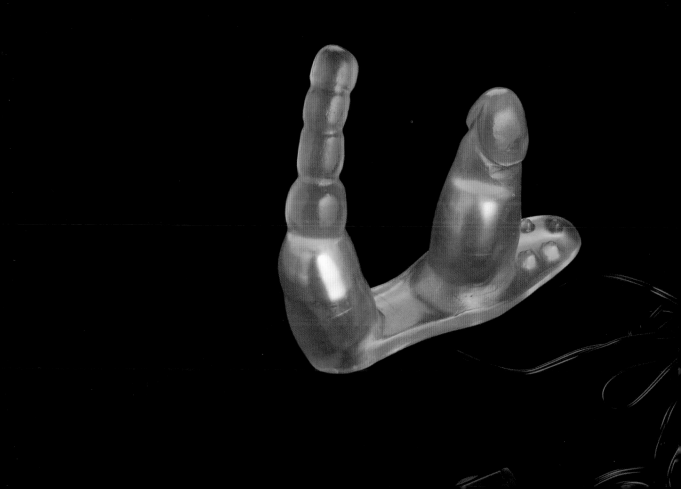

Shy

Appearance	●●●●●
Originality	●●●●●
Subtlety	●●●●●
Portability	●●●○○
Orgasmability	●●●●○

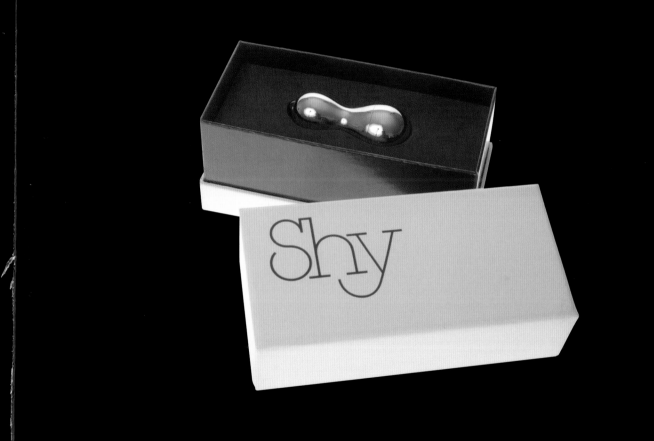

Ruby Thong

Appearance	○○○○○
Originality	●●●●○
Subtlety	●●○○○
Portability	●●●●○
Orgasmability	●●●○○

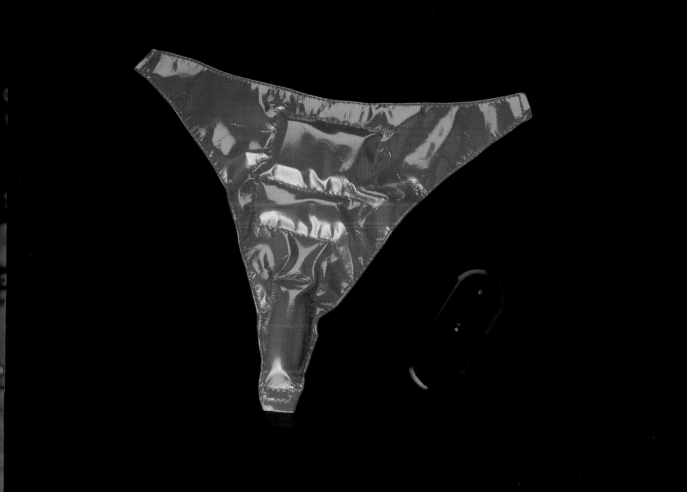

College Stud

Appearance	●●●●●
Originality	●○○○○
Subtlety	○○○○○
Portability	●○○○○
Orgasmability	●●●●●

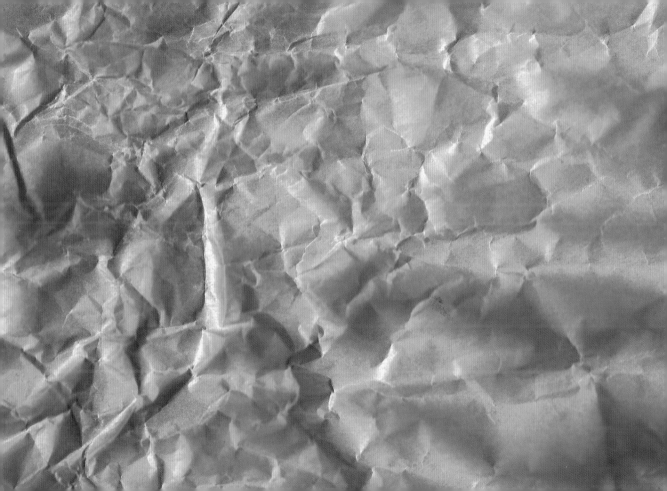

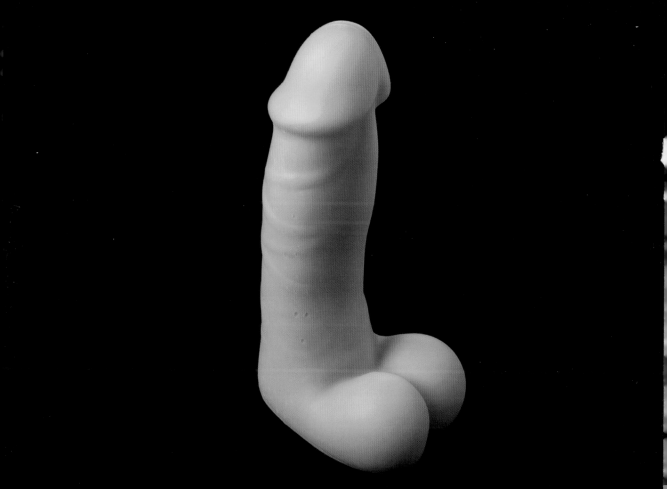

Index

The items photographed in this book were rigorously tested by a highly discerning panel of judges from the Scarlet team and kindly provided by the following retailers – if you would like to purchase any of these items then please contact the companies directly: Sextoys (www.SexToys.co.uk), Nice Sex toys (www.NiceSexToys.co.uk), Ann Summers (www.AnnSummers.com), Bedroom Pleasures (www.BedroomPleasures.co.uk), The Cone (www.ConeZone.org), Durex (www.Durex.co.uk/play), Lelo (www.Lelo.com), OhZone (www.OhZone.co.uk), Pink Pickle Toys (www.PinkPickleToys.com), Mates (www.Mates.co.uk), Shy (www.Shy-UK.com)

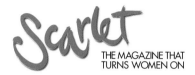

THE MAGAZINE THAT
TURNS WOMEN ON

Scarlet is packed with frank informative features that talk to the readers the way women talk to each other when men aren't around. *Scarlet* will never patronise or support tired stereotypes; men aren't all bastards, women can (and do) enjoy porn, and they don't all dream of being a size 10.

Scarlet's features are diverse, from the self-explanatory Worst Sex Tips Ever Written to cutting-edge articles like A Hand-Job By Any Other Name… reporting on the new craze of yoni (vulva) massage as a form of 'alternative therapy'.

Scarlet also comes with a **FREE** copy of Cliterature, a 30 page magazine crammed with hot erotic fiction and true confessions – every month!

To subscribe visit the website to see the latest deals:
www.ScarletMagazine.co.uk/100